TheReal Weight Loss Solution Handbook

10 Actions to Reshape Your Body, Mind and Spirit

Denise A. Brown
A VOICE FOR REAL HEALTH

I dedicate this book to all the brave souls who have tried and failed to overcome their weight issues, but who venture forward with hope to find their real weight loss solution.

Table of Contents

Acknowledgments

Beyond the hours I spent imagining and writing this book, there are other people who helped bring it to print. First, thanks go to my accountability partner, Chris Mahoney, for keeping me on track and sharing in great phone conversations. You are a friend for life and I look forward to reading your book which introduces the tasteful and worldly travels of Clarence Carrot. Next, thanks go to my son, Thomas Brown, for editing and proofreading my final draft. Thanks also go out to my daughter, Amber Damon, for being my sounding board through my frustrations and a guide in overcoming my anxiety with my lack of computer skills. A special thank you goes out to my hairdresser, Cindy Polley, who scheduled me in on short notice. She also took on the role as my photographer through her other business Cindy Polley Photography to provide a headshot for my book cover. Thanks are also extended to my many mentors. Thank you Joshua Rosenthal, founder of the Institute of Integrative Nutrition, for encouraging me to spread my message through this book. Thanks Lindsay Smith, instructor for the IIN Launch Your Dream Book course, for all the quotes and songs of inspiration and the know-how to get the job done. Thank you to all the experts- past and present IIN health coaches, hosts of online summits, and the doctors of Functional Medicine- all who freely share knowledge of alternatives to conventional health care practices. You have all helped me to obtain the knowledge shared within this book. Lastly, thanks go to my husband, Steve, for your patience and willingness to entertain yourself through all the time spent apart during the writing process.

Introduction

Our culture puts a lot of pressure on us to be thin. For many years television commercials have associated our life happiness with our weight. This is reinforced with the bombardment of ads for all sorts of weight reduction diet plans, special foods, intense workouts, weight loss drugs and even surgical procedures. And even though people have resorted to these measures for decades, we have the highest rate of obesity today and it is growing. It is obvious these strategies to control our weight are not working.

We know that it is hard for a lot of people to lose weight. There are many diets out there to try, but they fail to work for most. These diets tell us it is easy to lose weight if you just follow their plans. But even when you do, you can still experience failure. You think you did something wrong, and suffer with feelings of defeat. You are a victim, but you don't need to be.

In reality, there is no diet that will work for everyone. We are individuals with our own unique biochemistry. Our needs for nourishment, cognition and emotional support are based on this fact. At any given time, what is happening with your hormones, metabolism, nervous system, immune system, your muscles and bones, and even your gut microbiome, is unique to your body. Therefore, one diet strategy that works for you won't necessarily work for me.

So what can you do to lose weight? You can change your focus from your weight to your health. There is a saying that most people know. It is, "You are what you eat." This is often repeated in weight loss information. Although it says a lot, it doesn't say enough, because you are also what you think and what you feel. When trying to create change in your life, it is important to focus on your whole self. You may be wanting to change your body's appearance, but it also requires a change in your thoughts and emotions. You are a whole person and your body, mind and spirit all must be supported in order for any transformation to occur. You are a lot more than a number on a scale! Your weight is really a symptom of your lifestyle. This handbook was created with that in mind.

My own motivation for health and weight loss sent me on a journey. This book comes from the progress I made doing that work. It is not a prescription for an easy weight reduction program or a plan you simply follow to achieve weight loss. Instead it is a much different approach to your personal transformation. Whether you are a woman trying to lose weight after having a baby, a man trying to lose a "beer" belly, someone experiencing weight loss resistance and/or a growing muffin top rising above your favorite pair of jeans, the ideas presented are relevant to you. It is simply a handbook with actions you can take daily to get the results you hope for.

It is my wish that you can have the success that I now have. If you set your sights on a real goal, a true desire that drives you to do what you need to do, then you will reach your destination. Start by answering the question,"Why do I want to lose weight?" and then, "How do you see yourself when you do?" Use your answers to set your goal, commit totally to that goal, and get ready to take action. Use the following actions to get you moving on your journey as they light your way to a shapelier and healthier you!

Action #1 Show Yourself Love

The first thing you can do to transform your body is to learn to love it as it is. The easiest expression of love is a hug. It is a common practice for many people to express their love for another by giving them a hug. It is often an automatic response. Giving hugs to yourself can become automatic too. Just wrap your arms around your upper body and give a squeeze. It may seem awkward at first, but it can feel good or even great. Give it a try and see how it feels for you. If it helps you feel lighter, then every time you need a lift give yourself a hug. You can also add some words of affirmation such as,"I love you just the way you are" or "I love you". Always remember you deserve to love yourself no matter what!

Another version of this action is the Mirror Technique. This also may seem a bit awkward at first, but as you do it more and more, you feel better and better about yourself. You can use a full-length mirror or a handheld one. Use what you have. Position yourself directly in front of the mirror and look at your face. Let whatever thoughts you have come to you. If the thoughts are positive relish in them. If they are negative, this is your chance to change them. Look directly into your eyes in the mirror and say, "I love you just the way you are." Look deeply into your eyes and repeat.

Take this practice of self-love wherever you go. You can hug yourself anywhere and you can practice the Mirror Technique wherever there is a mirror. Or no matter where you are, you can always make the words, "I love myself just the way I am" your silent mantra. They are meant to help you accept yourself as you are, rather than how you wish to be.

Practice these affirmations often. The messages you give yourself are extremely important to being able to change. Your mindset determines the quality of your life and how much weight your body holds onto. If you do not love yourself fully, it will be harder to obtain and maintain a healthy, balanced body.

Action #2 Manage Your Stress

There is a lot of research that's focused on the effects of stress on your life and the ability to lose weight. Stress hormones stimulate you to seek out foods high in sugar, fat, salt, starches, or any combination of these. We already know how candy bars, potato chips, and ice cream can derail all weight loss efforts. Fortunately there is a practice that reduces stress, supports weight loss, and builds greater self-love. It is simply meditation.

Meditation relaxes your body and mind, and helps you get control over your thoughts by letting them just be. There are many different forms available on DVD, CD and through YouTube on the internet. One meditation form encourages you to visualize what you want, and another has you listen to sounds that change the way your brain functions. There are also methods that use hypnosis or breathing. All forms create a calm awareness and appreciation of yourself which can support your weight loss efforts. If you have headphones or earbuds and a quiet place to lay down or sit up undisturbed, you can have an incredible experience that can change your life forever.

If meditation seems too strange to you, there are other strategies you can use in order to manage your stress. For one, you can change the way you think about things. Your perception of your stress is key to how much stress you actually experience. So focus your thoughts on your pleasurable moments. Also, whenever you find yourself thinking negatively about something change those thoughts to positive ones. Another stress management tool is journaling. Writing down your feelings and thoughts about stressful events can help you look at these experiences in different ways, which can lead to emotional healing and personal growth. You can also plan for opportunities to have fun and laugh a lot. Laughing is a great stress buster. In addition, there are numerous deep breathing techniques available to help you relax and lower your levels of cortisol. The buildup of this stress hormone is known to increase appetite, interfere with the release of stomach acids, suppress the immune system, and increase incidences of depression and anxiety. It is extremely important to reduce cortisol levels to control weight and foster feelings of wellbeing.

Here is a simple breathing exercise you can use to calm your nervous system and your stressed out mind. You use a timed breath technique in which your exhale is longer than your inhale. Begin by closing your eyes and notice as you take a breath through your nose. Start your timed breathing by inhaling through your nose to a count of 4, hold for a count of 1, exhale for a count of 6, hold for a count of 1. Repeat for about five minutes. The length of your breath can be varied. Take breaths to a count that is comfortable for you.

Action #3 Get Enough Sleep

Sleep is necessary for a healthy body in so many ways. It is essential that you balance your day with rest to replenish your energy, rebuild your cells, reimagine your life and reconnect with yourself. It can help with your weight loss efforts and give your body a chance to repair daily wear and tear. You show yourself love by getting enough sleep.

Sleep is extremely important to your brain and your wellbeing. In fact some meditations create the same brainwaves as occur in sleep and is why it is a restorative practice. Throughout a day while awake you experience an incredible amount of information through your senses. Your brain is unable to process all this information until you sleep when this stimuli is sorted and stored in your brain as memories. Sleep is also the only time you get to dream. It is during the dream phase of sleep that calm is created in your mind.

It is important to have a consistent daily bedtime to get enough sleep. It is also beneficial to turn off electronics beforehand to help wind down before sleep. An ideal bedtime is 10:00 PM and a natural wake up around 7:00 AM. Although not everyone can follow the same time frames, it is most important to be consistent to optimize your health.

Your whole body requires adequate amounts of sleep to clear out the overload of toxins you are bombarded with every day in our present world. Interestingly, the glymphatic system has recently been discovered in our bodies. This is a drainage system that works while you sleep to clean out the garbage in your brain known as neurotoxins. So remember to show yourself love, you need to plan for and get around seven to nine hours of zzzs every night!

Action #4 Maximize Your Nutrition

It can be simple, but not necessarily easy. Eat real food and eat as much as you want so you're never hungry for junk food. When you eat plenty of real food such as vegetables, fruits, nuts and seeds, legumes, healthy fats, gluten-free grains, pastured eggs, wild-caught fish and grass-fed meats, your body gets the nourishment it needs. When you are nutritionally satisfied, you are no longer hungry. In contrast, when you eat processed (manmade) foods that lack in nutrient value, your body continues to look for nourishment and you remain hungry. There is no need to think you should count calories if you are eating real food.

Your body needs healthy fats. It is hard to know what those are though, because there is so much misinformation out there. For years we were told to stay away from all fats, but now we know that all fats are not created equal. There are some saturated, polyunsaturated, and monounsaturated fats that are beneficial. And yet there are others that are best to avoid. Some studies show the medium chain fatty acids (MCFAs) found in coconut oil support your health, while the trans fats like the shortening created by humans, don't. It is these hydrogenated oils, which are made by adding hydrogen to liquid vegetable oil to make it solid, that increase your risk of developing heart disease, stroke and type 2 diabetes. They are used in many processed foods and deep fried foods offered in regular and fast food restaurants. It is also important to understand the truth about cholesterol. Saturated fats do raise cholesterol, but cholesterol is NOT the cause of heart disease. However, our healthcare system still treats it as though it were. In fact, cholesterol is necessary for you to be healthy. Trust me on this or read The Great Cholesterol Myth by Dr. Stephen Sinatra and Jonny Bowden. Some fats that support your healthy body include coconut oil, extra virgin olive oil, avocado, and nuts and seeds. Canola oil is one fat that is promoted as a health food, but is much better to avoid.

Eat some sea salt every day. It is an essential nutrient and not the cause of hypertension as we were told. However, there are a few people who are identified as being salt-sensitive. Avoid using common table salt and processed foods high in sodium. Common table salt is a manmade product created through a refining process which depletes the essential nutrients that are naturally found in salt. During the processing chemicals are added like bleach, monosodium glutamate (MSG), and fluoride, which are all detrimental to your body. On the other hand, sea salt is a natural product. It comes from salt marshes, naturally occurring as the sun evaporates the water. No life-giving nutrients are lost with its harvest. It contains trace amounts of sodium, sulphur, potassium, calcium, magnesium, strontium, and silicon among others. Healthy people all over the globe consume about one and a half teaspoons a day. When consumed regularly it can reduce asthma symptoms, stabilize blood pressure, assist your brain in communicating with your muscles, and help your digestive system. Without it you will gradually perish. Eat some every day, just make sure it's the real kind.

Sugar is horrible for your body and it is necessary for it too. Your body needs sugar in the form of glucose to carry out different metabolic processes which provide you with energy. Fructose is one of the worst sources. Your body doesn't use it for energy, instead it goes directly to your liver and gets stored as fat. The sugar that is obtained through whole foods is the best source. Whole vegetables and fruit have fiber which helps the natural sugar in them release slowly into your bloodstream. This biological process provides energy without the fat storage. Try to get your sweet tooth satisfied with natural sugar foods.

Commit to eating a variety of real foods. Your body needs food that includes proteins, fats and carbohydrates. Although many diet plans suggest you need to greatly reduce or eliminate one of them, scientific studies show you actually need all three macronutrients every day to be healthy. You also need to eat food with many different micronutrients daily to live a balanced healthful life. Vitamins, minerals, enzymes, and probiotics are found in different foods. Eating a variety of foods daily will provide the various nutrients you need to have optimum health.

It is important to mention the need to feed your gut microbiome to maximize your nutrition. We have beneficial bacteria that live in our digestive tracts that help to break down our food into the nutrients our bodies need to keep us healthy. It is essential to support them by consuming probiotics in the form of fermented foods or pills. Some common probiotic foods and drinks include sauerkraut, kimchi, unpasteurized pickles, miso, kombucha, fermented coconut water, unpasteurized yogurt, and kefir. If you wish to use a supplement look for one with several strains of friendly bacteria and a resistance to acid and bile.

Strive to eliminate all processed foods from your diet. These food-like items are full of manmade ingredients that were never meant for human consumption. They are detrimental to your health, wellbeing and waistline, and are addictive too. Remember the line, "I bet you can't eat just one"? Enough said.

Go at your own pace in eliminating everything created in a laboratory. Think: genetically engineered (also known as GMO), sugar (high fructose corn syrup-HFCS), artificial sweeteners (aspartame, saccharin, sucralose), chemical flavorings (artificial vanilla) artificial colorings (petroleum-based Red 40), food preservatives (sodium nitrate), and other food additives (flavor enhancers, emulsifiers, thickening agents, binding agents, color carriers). Note: You will find lists for these categories in the Appendix.

Learning to make meals without processed foods can take time. Just try to avoid these foods as much as possible. Remember they can sabotage your weight loss efforts and set you up for a lot of disease in your body. As you eliminate more and more of these foods your body will thank you.

Action #5 Minimize Your Toxic Load

Today we are repeatedly exposed to many toxic substances. Our bodies have an amazing ability to handle a slew of insults, but in the present world we are under constant attack in our daily life. Our livers and kidneys do a great job cleaning out some of these poisons, but there is now too much for our innate detoxing systems to handle. Your body has a protective strategy to handle these excessive threats. It's called fat storage. The toxins that it is unable to handle at the present time gets stored in your fat cells. This is called visceral fat and it threatens your whole wellbeing. The more toxins you are exposed to, the more visceral fat storage occurs and weight loss becomes impossible. When you decrease the onslaught of toxins going into your body, in its innate wisdom, it will begin to release the poisons stored in your fat cells. Your body knows when it is able to rid itself of these hazardous substances and so becomes less resistant to weight loss.

You are what you ingest. Everything you put in your mouth affects you in some way. The food industry exists to sell you something. Often that something is a food-like item that contains many ingredients that are toxic to your body. If you wish to be healthy and have control over your weight, you need to eliminate processed foods from your diet. Of special note is the fact that pharmaceutical drugs prescribed by your doctor are also toxic to your body. These manmade substances are mostly used to treat symptoms your body is expressing. Unfortunately, the cause of what ails you is usually ignored and you are directed to take these drugs for an indefinite period of time. The longer you ingest a pharmaceutical the more likely you are to experience symptoms from the toxicity of that drug, and in turn are often prescribed another drug for those symptoms. You can end up taking many different drugs at one time that never address what was the cause of your original problem.

You are also exposed to substances in the toothpaste you use. Fluoride is a known neurotoxin—it effects your brain. If you wish to think clearly you need to eliminate fluoride toothpaste from your daily exposure. Aluminum-free baking soda is a safe substitute for toothpaste. (Aluminum is also toxic.) Or try this recipe for homemade toothpaste: Mix equal parts of coconut oil and baking soda, then add a few drops of tea tree oil and/or peppermint essential oil. Another substance that gets put in your mouth, but you don't swallow is dental silver fillings. These contain high levels of mercury, which is also a known neurotoxin. You are repeatedly exposed to this toxin every time you chew your food. If your dentist suggests you need a dental filling opt for the white kind.

You are what you absorb. Many of us forget that our skin is the largest organ of our body. Anything we put on the outside of us also effects our insides. If the ingredient in a product is a neurotoxin, whether ingested or absorbed, it can affect your brain. There are many known poisonous chemicals in our personal care products. One common one is propylene glycol (PG), an ingredient in antifreeze and also used as a preservative in deodorant, moisturizer, soap, shampoo, conditioner, eye makeup, aftershave lotion, and baby wipes. Note: It's also found in food and injectable drugs. Although the FDA has deemed it Generally Recognized As Safe (GRAS), the Material Safety Data Sheet calls it a hazardous substance and has handling instructions because contact with it can cause damage to skin, liver and kidneys. The Natural Health Center recommends using PG-free personal care products. Keep in mind that this is only one ingredient in these products that is toxic to your body.

Over time you can do some research on other chemicals found in your personal care items. Note: There are lists of known hazardous chemicals found in personal care products and household cleaning products in the Appendix.

You are what you inhale. Pollution is something we think involves factories spewing chemicals from smoke stacks and cities with smog. But the air in our homes is often full of toxins. You may be unknowingly polluting your home environment. Every time you burn a paraffin wax candle, spray an odor eliminator, or plug in an air freshener, you are contaminating the air you breathe. A paraffin wax candle is made with petroleum and when burning emits toxic soot into the atmosphere. Likewise, when you spray an odor eliminator or plug in an air freshener, you are releasing poisonous chemicals into your home. They all affect your body negatively and should be avoided. A good option for paraffin candles are beeswax candles. Chemical air fresheners can be replaced with essential oils or fresh fruits simmering in water. Remember there are always safer alternatives to the products advertised by the media.

You are also what you think and feel. We all experience toxic thoughts and feelings (anger, fear, hate) as givers and receivers. All negative thoughts you think or negative emotions you feel can shut down your ability to handle everyday life. You can learn coping skills to transform your toxic thoughts and feelings to positive energy that heals your body, mind and spirit. Learn to breathe deeply, set an intention to forgive and forget, and be grateful every day. By practicing these strategies to deal with the unavoidable stressors that occur as a regular part of life, you can reduce the negative, energy-zapping thoughts and feelings you have and those that come your way from others. Avoid excessive exposure to TV and other media with all their messages of doom and gloom, and feed your soul with positive life-affirming messages from inspirational leaders, mentors, and self-help gurus. Remember we all want to feel loved and appreciated. You can do this by supporting yourself and others with thoughts of love, compassion, kindness, and forgiveness.

Action #6 Shop, Cook and Eat Like a Chef

The first step to healthy eating is healthy shopping. Before you go shopping plan a menu (daily, weekly, or monthly), make a list to take with you, and eat or make sure you are not hungry beforehand. When you are at the store take time to shop for the best ingredients to support health.

Buy whole foods if possible. If you decide to use processed foods, be sure to read the labels on all cans, boxes and packages you are considering to buy. Many packaged frozen vegetables and canned legumes can be health promoting. They are usually minimally processed often with the particular food being the only ingredient. Read labels and avoid items with common salt added. Also remember to avoid hidden sugars and any poisonous (toxic) food additives. A general rule to follow is to buy packaged items that have less than three ingredients.

Whenever possible choose organic. The term "organic" means the food is grown and raised the way nature intended-- without genetically engineered organisms, poisonous pesticides, herbicides, synthetic fertilizers, and genetically engineered grain-feed. All organic eggs, meats, and dairy products are free of growth hormones and antibiotics. All of the animals raised for meat are grass-fed and pasture-raised. Remember you are what you eat. If you wish to be healthy, you will want to eat food that promotes health. Look in the Appendix for EWGs lists of The Dirtiest Dozen Plus and The Clean Fifteen.

After you've bought your ingredients then it's time to cook. There are so many healthy ways to prepare foods. You can boil, blanch, steam, stir-fry, sauté, grill or stew an assortment of ingredients on a stove top. Or maybe you would prefer to bake, broil or roast something tasty in the oven. Of course, you can always prepare some delicious cuisine on an outdoor barbecue. Pressure cookers and slow cookers (crock pots) are also great tools to use to prepare foods. Deep fat frying is one cooking method that is best to avoid. It is also advisable to avoid using nonstick surface pots and pans as your cooking tool.

No matter what cooking vessels you choose, it should be your goal to create satisfying tastes that touch all your tongue receptors. That is what chefs refer to as "a full-mouth taste". Unfortunately, many of us have had our taste buds warped by the food industry. By being encouraged to overconsume processed foods high in sweet and salty tastes, our taste for sour, bitter, pungent, and astringent have been seriously lacking. By gradually adding less familiar foods or foods cooked in different ways to your daily meals, you can train your palate to enjoy all flavors. The aroma wafting through your home of something delicious cooking in the oven can be a great way to get your digestive juices flowing. New taste sensations are just waiting to be created and enjoyed. Perhaps a cooking class is in your plans.

So once you know what to cook, how to cook those ingredients, and prepare your meal, it is time to eat. The presentation of the food on your plate along with the aroma from the preparation initiate the digestive response. It is also important to eat slowly and savor every bite of the healthy morsels you carefully prepare so you can get pleasure and nutritional satisfaction from your meal. Digestion starts in the mouth and so does your enjoyment of the food that nourishes your body, mind and spirit. Bon appetit!

Action #7 Get Support

Social support can help you achieve your health goals. While you work towards your desired outcomes, other people can hold you accountable and remind you of your goals. One or several people can help you make a lifestyle change a positive experience by supporting you emotionally while encouraging your new behaviors. It is always helpful to have someone to listen to you without offering advice, and who allows you to express your frustrations when they occur.

There are many people who can provide this support to you. Perhaps a family member, your spouse, a friend or a co-worker can help by celebrating your successes with you. You can seek out a mentor who serves as a model for your new behaviors. A mentor can also validate your feelings and offer you suggestions. If you are an emotional eater a counselor can offer support by providing ideas for regaining control of your eating habits. You could find a helper who can give you practical support by showing you new ways to prepare a food or helping you to learn how to read labels while you shop.

Or if you are looking for someone to do all these things and more, you could seek the help of an Integrative Nutrition Health Coach. This person is someone specially trained to emotionally support you as you set health goals and practice the behaviors necessary to reach them. A health coach helps you develop the confidence that is needed to create the lifestyle you desire and are determined to make your reality. An Integrative Nutrition Health Coach can provide a pat on the back and information you seek, offer emotional support, and is an accountability partner, a great listener, a role model, a comforting friend, and an all-around helper. Your health coach will provide the support you need to do the work that is necessary to reach your health goals.

Action #8 Move More, Sit Less

Movement is essential for a healthy body. Your body is biologically made to move. That's why sitting for extended periods of time can cause stiffness. Most of the exercises you are encouraged to do to help with your weight loss efforts, however, often put unnecessary stress on your body. Whenever we maintain an intense workout for an extended period of time as in cardio, we are encouraging our body to have a stress response. If you wish to practice this type of movement, you would be better off looking for some interval training exercises. These exercises reduce the time you are in an intense phase of movement, yet still allow your body to sweat.

There are other exercises that use gentle movements that stretch and nurture your body. Some great options are Yoga, Pilates, Tai Chi and Qigong. The slow deliberate movements of each of these practices are stress-free and soothing to your body, mind and spirit.

Things that get you moving that you enjoy are of greatest benefit to your health and wellbeing. Some choices include gardening, bouncing on a rebounder, taking a walk outside, or even standing while you do things that you would usually sit down for. Or perhaps you love to dance or would prefer to play a game of Red Light, Green Light with your kids. Whatever you choose, rejoice and be grateful you can move your amazing body.

Action #9 Practice, Practice, Practice

Repetition builds habits. It is common sense that it will take time to change your lifestyle habits. They were created over time and so will need time to change. The more you practice a new behavior, the more it will become a familiar one. Even this action of practice will become habit. You will gradually practice these actions without consciously acknowledging that you are. That is what a habit is. A habit is something you do without thinking about it. When you make all of these actions habits, you will then have habits that support your health and ability to lose weight rather than hinder them.

As you take a new action, go slow and give yourself time to adjust to your new behaviors and future life habits. Since it is the desire to lose weight that encouraged you to read about these actions, remind yourself that losing weight is part of being healthy and having a more vibrant life. You need to keep adding these actions to your daily life to get there, but you should do that at your own pace. Remember to make your new habits work for you. If you try to rush change, it can actually slow or stall your progress. As you slowly add and practice these actions you will recognize that you are truly a work in progress.

Action #10 Be Kind to Yourself

Ignore actions #2- 9. (You need to always love yourself to thrive- action #1.) Occasionally it's a great idea to throw the plan out the window. That bag of potato chips that's calling to you can be a great reminder of why you gave them up. The special birthday cake made for your child from his favorite boxed mix just may be what's needed to make his day truly special. You may feel the need to eat every bite of that very large expensive juicy steak. The idea is not perfection, but to celebrate your life and your health.

Accept your perfect imperfections. We are perfect as we are even with all of life's complications. You may have days when you have difficulty taking any action. Be kind to yourself and avoid the Blame Game or the Shame Game. Leave the torture tactics to someone else. Rejoice in being alive! No matter what happens!

Practice actions #1- 10. You can show yourself great love and kindness by taking action. Lip service doesn't change anything. Taking action does! Read through these actions and then decide to do them in any order you wish. Perhaps you'll choose to try several at once. It's not how you do it. It's that you DO do it! Your life is in your hands. Your health and wellbeing is your responsibility. By taking at least one of these actions you are accepting that responsibility and showing kindness to yourself.

Congratulate yourself on taking action #1. Being kind to yourself is another way to show yourself love!

Conclusion

Most of us are aware that we have an obesity epidemic and an increase in all chronic diseases in our country. What many people don't realize is that it is actually a global problem now as more and more countries adopt the American lifestyle. But in other areas in the world referred to as the Blue Zones, there are people who are lean, healthy and thriving. If we look away from our own culture and to these indigenous people in these zones there is much to learn.

They have lived and eaten the same way for thousands of years. They live the longest and healthiest lives of all people on the earth. You could assume that the solution to our obesity epidemic could be to eat like these other people, but that is too simple. As Americans we have access to a very large variety of food from all over the globe, even to some of the foods regularly eaten by these native cultures. What we can learn from these indigenous people is that true health comes from living in harmony with the earth and eating real foods grown with unadulterated soils and natural methods. When we replace all the foods we have grown and created with all our technological "advances", and go back to eating those grown with rich, naturally inoculated soils like these people, we can heal and thrive.

Over time we forgot how important it is to the earth and our own unique bodies to eat from our local food economies. These indigenous people have always eaten from their immediate environment. They have never had foods shipped to them from halfway around the world. Everything they eat is fresh and full of nutrients. The current population of these people also eat the same foods their ancestors ate and so they are well adapted to obtaining maximum nutrition from them. They also live in villages that support community connection and live in a way that honors the earth.

There are many things to consider when you are thinking about your health and weight. You need to consider your own individual genetics, your lifestyle, what you truly believe, how you feel about yourself, and you need to acknowledge what real foods and emotional support are available to you. It is only then that you can find the solution to your own health and weight problem.

Life is a journey with many things to learn along the way. Action must be taken daily to create the life you want. You may choose to see the struggles in your life you encounter as obstacles or opportunities. When you experience a failure with one diet approach, you can give up or you can try another. Life is made up of making many choices every day. Struggles that result in failures or successes are encountered regularly when you take any kind of action. The ability to keep going despite the outcome is necessary if you wish to be healthy and comfortable in your skin. You can begin by accepting responsibility for your own well-being. Then decide you are worth all the love you are more inclined to give another and give it to yourself first.

Your body is an amazing organism with the innate wisdom to carry you through a long healthy radiant life. The natural ability to stay strong and heal easily is presently challenged with all the toxins in our environment. You must accept that we have a lot of poor quality food available in the US. The actions you take to limit your exposure to them will determine whether your body survives or thrives. When you take responsibility for your health seriously and do the actions in this book, you will lose weight and thrive.

There are many more actions you can take besides what is in this book. For example, remembering to drink water throughout the day would be another beneficial action. However this book was purposefully kept small and simple so you could read it quickly. It also can be used as a resource you can take with you when you shop. The most important actions for you to take to obtain weight loss and create a happy and healthy you are the ones presented in this book.

Always remember to show yourself how much you care by what you allow to go into your inside, what you do to your outside, and finding others to share your amazing life with. It is when you do these things for yourself that you will find your real weight loss solution.

Appendix

A. GMOs, where they are found and how to avoid them

A genetically modified organism (GMO) of food is made by forcing the gene from one species into the DNA of a food crop to introduce a new trait. These foods are NOT real foods. They could never occur in a natural environment. That alone should tell you they are not able to support health. When you ingest foods with GMOs you are ingesting an artificial food. Health risks associated with the consumption of genetically engineered foods include infertility, immune problems, faulty insulin regulation, accelerated aging and changes in the major organs and the gastrointestinal system.

There are eight major GM food crops. They are corn, soybeans, sugar beets, canola, cottonseed, Hawaiian papaya, papaya from China, and some zucchini and yellow squash. Recently it was announced that GM potatoes and apples will soon be available in food stores. In America the sugar found in most processed foods is derived from GM sugar beets or a combination of sugar cane and GM sugar beets. Most dairy products come from cows injected with GM bovine growth hormone. There is also invisible GM ingredients in many processed foods (and personal care products). Most sources of sugars, artificial sweeteners and food additives have hidden GM sources unless they are organic or declared non-GMO.

Just knowing where GM ingredients and foods may be hiding can help you avoid them. Unfortunately at this time we do not have mandatory GMO labeling in the United States, although many states are trying to get the FDA to comply with the interest of the majority of Americans. The big corporations who manufacture these products are spending billions of dollars to fight this labeling and to confuse consumers about the independent scientific studies that show the detrimental effects of consuming and using GM products. Several tips you can use to avoid GMOs are: 1- buy organic, 2- look for Non-GMO project seals, and 3- avoid at-risk ingredients and processed foods. You can also join the fight to get these products labeled.

B. The numerous and often hidden names of sugar

Look for the –ose suffix word ending to identify sugars in processed foods. These include dextrose, fructose, galactose, glucose, lactose, maltose, mannose, pentose, saccharose, sucrose, and zylose.

Other names for sugar include; agave, agave nectar, anhydrous dextrose, Barbados sugar, barley malt, barley syrup, beet sugar, blackstrap molasses, brown rice syrup, brown sugar, buttered sugar, buttered syrup, cane juice, cane juice crystals, cane juice solids, cane sugar, caramel, carbitol, carob syrup, castor sugar, coconut sugar, concentrated fruit juice, confectioner's sugar, corn sweetener, corn syrup, corn syrup solids, crystal dextrose, crystalline fructose, date sugar, datem, dehydrated cane juice, dehydrated fruit juice, demera sugar, dextran, dextrin, diatase, diatastic malt, diglycerides, disaccharides, erythritol, ethyl maltol, evaporated cane juice, Florida crystals, free-flowing brown sugars, fructooligosacchrides, fructose sweetener, fruit juice, fruit juice concentrate, fruit juice crystals, fruit juice solids, fruit juice syrup, glucitol, glucoamine, glucose solids, golden sugar, golden syrup, granulated sugar, grape sugar, hexitol, high fructose corn syrup (HFCS), honey, icing sugar, inversol, invert sugar, isomalt, lakanto, liquid fructose, maltodextrin, malted barley, malts, malt syrup, mannitol, maple syrup, molasses, molasses syrup, muscavado sugar, nectars, organic raw sugar, oat syrup, palm sugar, pancake syrup, panela, panocha, powdered sugar, raisin syrup, raw sugar, refiner's syrup, ribose rice syrup, rice bran syrup, rice malt, rice syrup, rice syrup solids, sorbitol, sorghum, sorghum syrup, stevia, sucanat, sucanet, sugar, sweet sorghum, syrup, tapioca syrup, treacle, turbinado, turbinado sugar, yellow sugar, white sugar, xylitol, and 100% fruit juice.

C. The names of artificial sweeteners

Acesulfame Potassium (ACE, Ace K, Acesulfame K) contains methylene chloride a known carcinogen. The brand names for this chemical are Sunnett, Sweet One, Sweet & Safe.

Advantame (GMO) is a newly approved artificial sweetener and derivative of Aspartame.

Alitame is found in many processed foods, but is not approved in the US.

Aspartame (GMO) is in a vast amount of processed foods. There are over 10,000 documented reports made to the FDA of adverse reactions to this brain poison. Two common brand names are NutraSweet and Equal.

Cyclamate (calcium cyclamate, cyclamic acid) is a chemical that was banned in US in 1970, but is approved in many other countries.

Erythritol (GMO unless certified organic) occurs naturally in some fruits, but most is produced by fermenting the sugar in corn with yeast.

Isomalt (GMO) is a sugar alcohol manufactured from GMO sugar beets.

Lactitol (GMO unless certified organic) is sugar alcohol manufactured from the milk of cows more commonly fed GMO corn. It is never suitable for someone with lactose intolerance or a dairy allergy.

Maltitol (GMO unless certified organic) is a sugar alcohol that comes from corn or wheat.

Mannitol (GMO) is a sugar alcohol derived from the fructose in GMO corn and is not well absorbed by the body. In excessive amounts it can have a laxative effect.

Neotame (GMO) is another derivative of Aspartame used in small quantities that exclude it from the ingredient list requirement set by the FDA. However, it can be found on labels listed as E961.

Saccharin (GMO) is a sulfa-based sweetener that is banned in other countries, but not the US. It is shown to cause cancer of the urinary tract, bladder, uterus, ovaries, blood vessels, and other organs of rodents in numerous lab studies. The diet food industry put pressure on the US and Canadian governments and this artificial sweetener is now approved without any warnings. The Center for Science in the Public Interest recommends avoiding this chemical found in Sweet'n'Low.

Sucralose (GMO) is created by chlorinating sugar. By adding three chlorine molecules to one molecule of sugar the chemical created is almost identical to the now banned pesticide DDT. It is found in Splenda.

Xylitol (GMO unless certified organic) is a sugar alcohol found in fruits and vegetables, but mostly made from GMO corn. It can cause gastrointestinal issues.

D. Some other food additives (Chemical flavorings, artificial colors, food preservatives, etc.)

Ammonium Carbonate is used as a leavening agent in baked goods, and is an ingredient in baking powder. It is on the Right to Know Hazardous Substance List. Inhaling ammonium carbonate can irritate the nose, throat, and lungs, and it can also irritate the skin and eyes.

Amyl Acetate is extracted pear and banana oils used to create artificial flavors. This chemical may cause indigestion, chest pain, headaches, fatigue, depression, and can irritate the mucus membranes. Other artificial flavorings have been linked to allergic and behavioral reactions.

Annatto bixin is a yellow orange food coloring used in cheddar cheese that is extracted from the seed coats of the tropical tree Bixa orellano. It has been linked to food-related allergies.

Benzoate (BHT, BHA, TBHQ) is used to preserve fats and prevent them from going rancid. This chemical can cause hyperactivity, allergies, skin rashes, asthma, dermatitis, tinnitus, tumors, nausea, vomiting, and affect estrogen levels. It is being looked at as a cause of brain damage and as a carcinogen.

Benzyl Acetate is related to Amyl Acetate. It can cause considerable discomfort as an irritant to the respiratory and intestinal tracts.

Bromated vegetable oils (BVO) is a chemical that enhances the flavor in many citric-based fruit juices and sodas. This additive can damage the liver, kidneys, testicles, heart and thyroid.

Canthaxanthin is a red-orange food dye fed to farmed salmon to make their flesh look more like wild salmon. It is also found in sunless tanning products. It has been linked to hepatitis, skin surface damage and impaired digestive system.

Caramel is a common flavoring and coloring agent that can cause Vitamin B6 deficiency.

Diacetyl is a butter flavoring found in butter, butterscotch, and butter-flavored popcorn. It is responsible for the rare and serious lung disease known as "Popcorn Workers Lung".

High fructose corn syrup (HFCS) is a cheap sugar alternative used to preserve freshness in baked goods and sweeten many processed foods. It increases your risk for type 2 diabetes, coronary heart disease, stroke, and cancer, and causes metabolic issues in your liver which lead to obesity, insulin resistance, and increased belly fat.

Monosodium glutamate (MSG) is used as a flavor enhancer in many processed foods and Chinese restaurant items. It can stimulate your appetite and cause headaches, nausea, wheezing, edema, a change in heart rate, difficulty breathing and burning sensations.

Olestra/ Olean is a fat substitute used in commercial fried and baked foods. It inhibits the absorption of some nutrients and has been linked to gastrointestinal issues.

Phosphates are added to processed foods as preservatives, emulsifying agents, acidifying agents, acidity buffers, and flavor enhancers. High usage of products with phosphates are linked to chronic renal failure and cardiovascular disease.

Potassium Bromate is an oxidating agent used in the process of making commercial bread. It is a known carcinogen with evidence of development of cell tumors in the kidneys and thyroid. It has been banned for use in food products in Europe and Canada.

Potassium Sorbate is a food preservative that has been linked to allergic reactions, nausea, diarrhea, and DNA damage.

Propyl Gallate is used as an artificial food preservative used to prevent oils from going rancid. It can be found in meat products, microwaveable popcorn, soup mixes, frozen meals, and mayonnaise. It is also added to cosmetics and pharmaceuticals. It may cause cancer, kidney, liver and respiratory problems and has been shown to cause stomach and skin irritation. It is banned in other countries.

Propyl Paraben is a derivative of benzoic acid and is used as a preservative and flavoring in foods, pharmaceuticals, and personal care products to extend shelf life. Parabens act as estrogen mimics and are potential endocrine system disruptors.

Red Dye 40 is a food colorant known to cause numerous neurological issues including ADHD, OCD and ODD. It has also been linked to certain birth defects and cancer. Other food colorings have been linked to allergies, sinus congestion and worsening symptoms of hyperactivity attention issues in children.

Sodium Benzoate is a preservative that is converted to benzene when it is heated and is in the presence of Vitamin C. It is found in fruit juices, jellies and jams that have fruits high in this vitamin. Benzene is known to damage DNA and to be a carcinogen.

Sodium Nitrate and Nitrite are used to preserve, color, and flavor cured meats and fish. They can combine with other chemicals in the stomach to form a known carcinogen. They are known to cause allergic reactions.

Sulfites are also used as preservatives. They are known to cause allergic reactions, especially in asthmatics.

Vanillan is an artificial vanilla flavorant sourced from the waste of paper mills and petroleum processing. It can cause allergic reactions and can significantly reduce the release of dopamine in the liver.

E. Hazardous chemicals found in household products & environmental chemicals

There are many chemicals that are referred to as Obesogens. They are a class of chemicals that have the ability to interfere with fat metabolism and cause fat accumulation particularly in the abdominal region of the body. Many of the following chemicals are obesogens.

Ammonia is a strong colorless gas used in cleaning products. It can release a highly toxic and possible deadly gas when mixed with bleach. On its own it is an irritant to skin, eyes, and lungs and in large amounts it is a poison.

Atrazine is a common herbicide used on corn crops in the US that is found in 94% of our drinking water. This chemical causes mitochondrial dysfunction which leads to insulin resistance and increased belly fat and body weight.

Chlorine is a highly reactive gas. It can irritate the skin, eyes and lungs when breathed in for a short amount of time. Repeat exposure to chlorine in the air can affect the immune system, the blood, the heart and the respiratory system. Chlorine harms the environment at low levels.

Dioxins are chemical contaminants usually found in soil and occasionally in water and air. People are more likely to be exposed by eating food contaminated with dioxins. It can accumulate in fatty tissues and people exposed to high levels are at great risk for cancer, reproductive and development problems, heart disease and diabetes.

Flame retardants can present health concerns. Organohalogen and organophosphorus pose health and environmental impacts. They are considered Persistent Organic Pollutants (POPs) since they do not break down into safer chemicals, they travel far from the source of release, they accumulate in the tissues of humans and other animals, and they are toxic. They are associated with endocrine and reproductive issues, immune and neurological system impairment and cancer.

Formaldehyde is found in spray and wick deodorizers and is a suspected carcinogen.

Glycol ethers are derived from crude oil and are used in paints, perfumes, liquid housecleaning soaps, and cosmetics. They are especially hazardous to your lungs and skin. Short term exposure to high levels of these solvents can cause severe liver and kidney damage and can result in pulmonary edema and narcosis. Long term exposure can cause nausea, fatigue, anemia, and tremor.

Heavy metals can be toxic. Lead, cadmium, mercury, and aluminum can damage our blood, kidneys, lungs, liver and other organs. Toxic exposure can result in reduced central nervous system function, mental impairments, and low energy levels. Zinc is beneficial at low levels, but is toxic at high doses.

Perchlorate is a chemical that can affect thyroid function at high doses. It is used to produce rocket fuel, fireworks, flares, and explosives and is found in plastic wrap, batteries, fertilizers, milk and produce. The FDA monitors levels of this chemical in our food. It is a known toxin to the thyroid gland, metabolism, and hormonal balance. It is also harmful to the environment.

Perflurochemicals (PFOA) are used to make products resistant to water, heat, oil and grease in the body or in the environment. They are found in nonstick cookware, food packaging and carpeting. They are thyroid disruptors that interrupt normal metabolic processes and interfere in the production of leptin the hormone that regulates appetite and weight control.

Phthalates and Bisphenols are chemicals used as solvents and fixatives to set color and scent. They are found in plastic products such as storage containers, food packaging, children's toys, detergents, and personal care products including nail polish and shampoo. These chemicals in low concentrations cause disruptions in metabolism, hormone regulation, reproduction, thyroid function, immunity, neurologic function and fetal development. They are directly linked to obesity and insulin resistance.

Phosphates are chemical compounds containing phosphorus. They are used in automatic dish detergents to remove grease, oil, and soil, and help to soften water and prevent spotting and buildup of film on dishes. They have been banned from laundry detergent in the US since the 1990s, but are still found in other cleaning products. Phosphates pose a great risk to the fish and plants in our lakes and streams. They also cause rashes, dizziness, and scratchy throats in those using cleaning products with phosphate. Processed foods with large amounts of phosphate can cause lung cancer and affect kidney and heart function.

Sodium Lauryl Sulfate is a common ingredient in personal care products that allows foam to form. Although it is obtained from coconuts, it is made toxic during the manufacturing process. It is linked to cancer, neurotoxicity, organ toxicity, skin irritation, and endocrine disruption.

Triclosan and Triclocarban are antimicrobials added to common household products such as soap, deodorant, toothpaste, socks, lunchboxes and countertops. They can be absorbed through the skin and can lead to resistant strains of bacteria as well as adverse changes in endocrine and reproductive systems and thyroid function. Soap and water are safer and green cleaners.

F. Environmental Working Group's (EWGs) Dirty Dozen Plus and Clean Fifteen Lists- these lists can assist you as you move your diet from one high in toxins to one that is brimming with maximum nutrition.

*These conventionally grown foods tested at the highest levels of pesticide residues.

1- apples 2- strawberries 3- grapes 4- celery

5- peaches 6- spinach 7- sweet bell peppers

 8- nectarines 9- cucumbers 10- cherry tomatoes

11- imported snap peas 12- potatoes 13- hot peppers

14- kale/ collard greens

*These conventionally grown foods tested at the lowest levels of pesticide residues.

1- avocados 2- sweet corn 3- pineapple 4- cabbage

5- frozen sweet peas 6- onions 7- asparagus

8- mangoes 9- papayas 10- kiwi 11- eggplant

12- grapefruit 13- cantaloupe 14- cauliflower

15- sweet potatoes